Bulletproof Diet

Heal Your Body And Transform It Into A Fat-burning
Machine For Optimal Weight Loss

(Start Your Low- Carb Diet Voyage With Simple And
Budget-Friendly Meals)

Tommy Castonguay

TABLE OF CONTENT

Chapter 1: Differences Between The Ketogenic Diet And The Atkins Diet

Even in the final phase of the Atkins diet, the keto and Atkins diets both restrict carbohydrate consumption. However, there are important distinctions.

Restriction

The Atkn diet permits moderate roe consumption. The ketogenic diet is significantly more restrictive than the Atkins diet.

The ketogenic diet places a greater emphasis on carbohydrate elimination and restricts the body's ability to convert protein into glucose for energy.

The vast majority of calories on the ketogenic diet are derived from fat.

The Atkins diet initially restricts carbohydrate consumption while permitting moderate protein consumption. As the journey progresses, the Atkn diet becomes more relaxed, allowing for more meat and a wider variety of foods.

Ketosis

Both the ketogenic and Atkins diets result in ketosis.

On the Atkins diet, however, only the first and sometimes second stages involve the carbohydrate restriction necessary to maintain ketosis. If a person follows the keto diet protocol, the ketosis will continue.

enduring viability

No robust, long-term studies indicate that restrictive, low-carbohydrate diets are healthy over the long term. In speed, the inverse may be true.

Research conducted on In 202 8, the Lancet Public Health found an increased risk of mortality among individuals consuming a low-carbohydrate diet high in animal protein and fat.

The researchers also discovered that individuals consuming a diet limited in saturated fat and protein had a reduced risk of mortality. Many of these whole grains, nuts, and legumes also contain dietary fiber. As a result, you are highly restricted to a low-salt diet.

Some individuals find the Atkins diet to be an achievable long-term option. As a person gets closer to their target weight, they increase their consumption of food and carbohydrates.

The final phase, or maintenance phase, of the Atkins diet may feel more manageable than sticking with the perpetually restrictive ketogenic diet. However, staying in ketosis for an extended period of time is hazardous. In addition, most reptiles are unable to sustain a very high fat intake or extreme sarb restriction for an extended period of time.

Origins

In the 2 920s, doctors developed the ketogenic diet to treat erleru.

Researchers have noted that it may have additional benefits, and since the mid-2 990s, the diet has become more prevalent.

Dr. Robert Atkins created the Atkins diet as a simple, low-carbohydrate nutritional approach. The roster has changed over the years to accommodate its four-stage structure.

Developing Healthy Eating Habits

Selecting an eating pattern that satisfies the individual's nutrient requirements over time

Account for all consumed foods and beverages and determine how they fall into the eating schedule.

Follow food safety guidelines when preparing food to reduce the risk of foodborne illnesses.

The purpose of this book is to provide a concise diet plan for those who wish to monitor their weight as well as their nutritional intake. Diet and inactivity are the primary contributors to a rotund generation. Without physical activity, it is possible to contract cardiovascular diseases, hypertension, osteoporosis, and other common ailments.

Recent surveys indicate that up to 2 10 percent of American households lack the financial means to acquire the proper food and, consequently, nutrition. Other segments of the population, despite being able to afford a full supper, consume less of what they should if compared to the recommended levels of intake.

The documentation of this type of diet places a significant emphasis on children because their stage in the development of the adult male is crucial in every aspect. In addition, the majority of chronic disease risk factors have begun to manifest in younger age groups. It is also common for individuals to maintain their eating habits well into their senior years, easily making the early interruption of these habits a top priority.

Chapter 2: The Significant Burden Of Diet-Related Chronic Diseases

Approximately 6 7% of the population is affected by cardiovascular disease. Tobacco use, hypertension, type 2 diabetes, and obesity are the primary risk factors for the maladies.

6 8 % of U.S. adults suffer from hypertension. It is a significant risk factor for cardiovascular disease, stroke, heart failure, and kidney disease. Approximately 2 6% of Americans are at risk for prehypertension.

Diabetes – In the United States, approximately 2 2 % of the population has diabetes, while approximately 6 10 % are in the prediabetic stage. This is a stage in which the blood sugar levels are slightly higher than normal, but not high enough to qualify as diabetes.

However, it should be emphasized that the age group afflicted the most by the diabetes statistics is those over the age of 20.

Nearly one in two men and women will eventually be diagnosed with cancer, according to research. This translates to approximately 8 2   percent of the population.

Osteoporosis - Osteoporosis will affect one out of every two men and one out of every four men in their lifetime. This statistic pertains to males over the age of 10 0. Approximately 80% of a girl's bone mass is acquired at the age of 2 8, whereas a boy's is acquired at the age of 20.

The book is divided into the following chapters:

The factors associated with calorie balance and obesity are described. It also discusses diet and exercises in relation to the individual's physique.

Reduced Foods and Food Components: this section is devoted to the food components that Americans consume in excess of the recommended quantities.

Increased Foods and Nutrients Include: This section discusses the nutrients that one should incorporate into their chosen diet. This includes fat-free and low-milk foods, as well as those abundant in potassium, as previously stated.

Creating a Healthy Eating Pattern entails combining the nutrition recommendations into a consistent pattern that must be followed by the individual desiring to develop improved nutrition patterns.

Helping People Easy make Healthier Decisions: The ultimate purpose of this book is to direct the American towards the optimal nutrition pattern for his or her occupation. This facilitates even the adoption of the optimally nutritious diet by future generations. This phase, however, must be carried out in the most remote areas where the average American may reside.

This book's material and content are applicable to and can be utilized by a variety of government agencies and departments devoted to the welfare of society. This includes educational institutions, health institutions, and even religious institutions, as most, if not all, religions value the purity of the body in addition to the purity of the spirit.

Our understanding of nutrition continues to expand, but surprisingly, our dietary habits do not appear to have changed in the intervening time. More than ever before, consumers in the modern era require sensible and professional advice regarding the type and composition of their meals.

Consequently, the primary objective for a nation with a healthy eating schedule is to target the youthful population before anything else. This creates a welcome foundation not only for the future, but also for the present, as dietary patterns among the younger generation are certain to spread as rapidly as was previously conceivable.

Maintaining a healthful diet is also relative to the population subgroup. For instance,

Before becoming expectant, it is essential for women to maintain a healthy and balanced weight. This is necessary so that they can avoid the dangers of pregnancy-related complications.

Pregnant women are encouraged to acquire weight, but within a professional-determined limit. Pregnant women may face a health risk if their weight gain exceeds the acceptable range.

Adults aged 610 or older are prohibited from engaging in activities that contribute to weight gain, as weight loss at this stage is advantageous for the individual.

In developed nations, the prevalence of obesity can be attributed to environmental factors that influence weight gain. In the modern workplace, for instance, there are more food outlets, which makes it more convenient for customers to choose from a variety of items. The consumer typically evaluates the nutritional value of these products based on their flavor. Such environments encourage excessive calorie consumption and limited physical activity.

It is important to observe that the average consumption, or rather the average number of calories available in the average American diet, has increased by approximately 600 calories over the past several decades. There has been an increase in portion sizes, and research indicates that what is currently served is extremely high in caloric.

It has been discovered that communities with more fast food restaurants have a higher BMI rate than those with fewer. It has been documented that, compared to the 2 970s, the number of fast food chains in the twenty-first century has multiplied. This has proved to be problematic for Americans' food choices. It has been found, for instance, that a greater proportion of people dine out than in previous generations. Older generations' sedentary natures and sedentary behaviors have ingrained a culture of eating away from home in young adults and children, which is a result of their sedentary natures and behaviors. The majority of Americans engage in less physical activity than they did in previous decades due primarily to changes in the workplace and the transition in cultures, including the eating culture.

Since the majority of the population consumes calorie-dense foods in excess of the recommended consumption, there has been a significant increase in the number of cases of obesity reported in the country. Men and women older than 2 9 tend to consume 2,68 0 and 2 ,7810 calories on average, respectively. Despite the fact that this number may not appear to be excessive or hazardous, it is important to note that many participants in studies such as this tend to provide inaccurate responses to protect their privacy and self-esteem.

Chapter 3: Tips For A Muscle Gain Diet Based On The Best Nutrition For Muscle Growth

In order to increase muscle mass, it is essential to consume foods that provide the optimal nutrients for muscle growth. This is nearly as essential as regular gym attendance.

If you do not consume the proper nutrients for gaining muscle, your intense training will yield fewer results. If you are underweight and have difficulty gaining weight, it is especially essential for you to track the nutrition you receive from your food.

My Six Nutritional Tips For Muscle Gain:

Consume Food Every 2.10 - 6 Hours

A meal every three hours is beneficial for those who want to gain muscle, those who want to eliminate fat and gain muscle, and those who want to gain muscle alone. Skipping meals to lose weight is not a good idea, as your body may begin to store fat as a protective mechanism.

Because it speeds up the body's metabolism, eating more frequently facilitates weight loss. If you can't gain weight readily, it's crucial that you eat every 6 hours or so, because if you don't, your body won't have a constant energy source and it may start consuming muscle tissue for the energy it needs, which prevents muscles from growing.

To Grow, Your Muscles Need Protein.

Meat, eggs, cheese, quinoa, legumes, tuna, salmon, cod, and peas are protein-rich examples of foods. Your recommended daily protein intake is approximately 2 .10 grams per pound of bodyweight (6   .6   grams per kilogram).Every meal should contain 8 0-60 grams of protein.

Protein is an essential building block for muscles, and it accelerates muscle recovery. If you wish to use a protein powder supplement, it should not exceed 8 0 percent of your daily protein intake. This is to ensure that your diet contains sufficient minerals, vitamins, and digestive enzymes.

Carbohydrates are essential to a healthy diet

Simple (sugars), complex (whole-grain cereals, brown rice), and fibrous (vegetables) are the three categories of carbohydrates.Concentrate on complex carbohydrates when exercising intensely and gaining muscle, as they release energy more slowly and for a longer duration.

Complex carbohydrate-rich foods include, among others, whole cereals, cornmeal, bran, pasta, and brown rice. You should consume the majority of your carbohydrates in the morning and after exercise. A nutritious meal following exercise is essential for muscle growth and recuperation.

Your daily carbohydrate intake should be approximately 10 .10 g per kilogram of bodyweight (2.10 g per pound).

Veggies Are Important

Every meal should contain 2 -2 glasses of fruits and vegetables. Fruits and vegetables contain anti-oxidants, vitamins, and minerals, which accelerate muscle recovery and repair damaged muscle cells.

High acid loads in the blood, created by cereals and proteins, must be neutralized with alkaline-rich vegetables and fruits. Too much acid in the blood can lead to a decrease in bone density and muscle mass.

Fat is also essential

Depending on whether or not you wish to lose body fat, 2 0-6 0% of your meal should consist of fat. Those who do not gain weight easily should have 6 0 percent body fat, those who would like to lose weight should have 2 0 percent, and the remainder should have 20 percent.

Consuming fat is essential for the body, and among its many benefits are its contribution to energy and oxygen diffusion in the circulation. Some foods that contain "good fat" (essential fatty acids) include olive oil, hazelnuts, seafood, and pumpkin seeds.

Record What You Consume

Keep a record of what and when you consume in order to keep track of the food you are consuming and whether it is beneficial to your muscle-building efforts. Gather information about each meal, including its nutritional value and the quantity of fat, carbohydrates, and protein consumed.

Even if this doesn't sound particularly enjoyable, it quickly becomes routine and has numerous advantages. If you often neglect to eat, you could set your phone to alert you when it is time to eat.

How to Get Going

Any transition can be difficult. From eating at a novel restaurant to consuming a variety of foods. It makes no difference if you are attempting to lose weight, feel fantastic, or simply want to kick ass. It gets worse when you have no idea where to begin. I'm about to simplify things for you. It is preferable to complete the stages sequentially, but don't be too hard on yourself if you can't.

Most individuals believe they have failed if they do not eat perfectly. So they just resolve to quit. This is a terrible suggestion. The benefit of this diet is that it does not require strict adherence.

The Bulletproof regimen is unlike any other regimen currently on the market. Many people wonder if it will still work if you don't follow the principles and consume non-organic vegetables or the proper meat and seafood. The simple answer is absolutely. The more you can perform successfully, the better off you will be.

You can become stronger and healthier by easily making minor adjustments. For some, this may involve creating a checklist. You will be presented with a guide for transitioning from a standard diet to the Bulletproof diet. Changes such as exercise will not be covered in this guide, as the emphasis will be on eating patterns. When you are juggling a job, a family, and activities that easy make life enjoyable, an information excess can be problematic. Consequently, we will examine dietary modifications as the first measure.

The steps are cumulative, so the more you accomplish, the better you will become. Take the initial measure and proceed. It can be intimidating to determine what to eat given the abundance of information available.

2 8 Essential Steps to the Bulletproof Diet

Easy cut out sweets. This includes all fruit liquids and beverages containing agave, honey, or high fructose corn syrup.

Consume calories from nutritious lipids. Use grass-fed butter, ghee, coconut oil, Upgraded XCT oil, or Brain Octane.

Eliminate all gluten. This refers to cereal, pasta, and bread. Do not consume gluten-free junk cuisine.

Get rid of vegetable oil, grain derived oil, and grains in general. This consists of canola, soybeans, and maize. Eliminate all polyunsaturated oils, such as peanut, flax, and walnut oil.

Stop consuming artificial flavors, colors, and additives. This includes synthetic flavors, colors, MSG, and aspartame.

Consume copious quantities of grass-fed meats from animals such as bison, lamb, and cattle. This dish pairs well with crustaceans, eggs, and fish.

Remove legumes such as lentils, beans, and peanuts. If you have no choice but to ingest them, you must soak, ferment, and cook them first.

Stop imbibing homogenized, pasteurized, and processed dairy products. It is acceptable to pasteurize high-fat foods, but they must be grass-fed. Some individuals may be able to consume grass-fed cows' fresh, whole, full-fat milk.

Start consuming wild seafood and livestock raised on grass. Consume free-range eggs, duck, poultry, pork, and chicken.

Consume only organic fruits and vegetables.

Cook with care, if at all. If possible, cook with water and at very low temperatures. No frying or microwaving allowed.

Do not consume more than one or two fruit servings per day. Instead of apples and cantaloupe, consume only low-fructose fruits like lemons or berries.

Utilize seasonings. rosemary and thyme are superior to granules. Use only recently opened, high-quality spices.

Enjoy your meals!

Key Considerations to Keep in Mind

If you must consume any form of fake, junk, or cheat food, do so. Do not tear yourself up and consider yourself a failure. The further you stray from the Bulletproof Diet, the fewer results you will see. The greater your efforts, the greater your rewards. Variations are acceptable and do not indicate failure.

If you develop acne, an allergy, or any other adverse effect after consuming dairy, use only ghee as your dairy source. Consume coconut oil and meat fat.

Do not count calories in an attempt to lose weight. Eat until satiated, then cease.

Avoid snacking. Intermittent fasting is encouraged, but not required.

Keeping your fruit consumption to one or two servings per day will help you avoid high triglycerides. The remaining reasons to limit your consumption are not fatal.

A diet abundant in healthy fats is required. You should consume 2 0 to 6 0 percent protein, 10 to 6 0 percent carbohydrates, and 10 0 to 80 percent fat.

Consume the least quantity of polyunsaturated fat possible. Use krill and fish oil supplements if you do not consume salmon weekly.

If it is difficult to locate grass-fed meats, choose the leanest grain-fed meat. When purchasing grass-fed meat, choose the fatty portions.

Do not use a lack of time as an excuse. The preparation of Bulletproof Coffee and soft-boiled eggs takes little time. Maintaining a healthy body and psyche is not optional. It is essential.

If you can do this reasonably well, you will live a life of high vitality, high performance, and low inflammation.

Chapter 4: First and foremost, what exactly is the failsafe diet?

The bulletproof diet was created by a man who was sick and tired of attempting countless different diets and enrolling in thousands of exercise programs, only to return to his original condition of being overweight, exhausted, and lethargic. He began researching these various diet plans and modified some of their steps while keeping track of how they affected his body. This individual used the scientific method to find a solution to his problem, and when all was said and done, he realized that his issue was simply inflammation. Yes, irritation! His entire body was inflamed, and this inflammation manifested itself in numerous ways. Because his brain was inflamed, he would study diligently for tests but fail miserably, he would walk short distances and develop blisters on his feet because his body was inflamed, and he would try all of these various dieting techniques but still remain overweight. Because chronic inflammation is the underlying cause of the majority of health-related maladies that are prevalent today, I believe it is imperative that I explain inflammation in detail. Alzheimer's, cancer, and heart disease are all caused by inflammation, which also contributes to the development of hundreds of other diseases.

Inflammation

Inflammation is the body's protective response to an invasion of pathogens, irritants, or other detrimental stimuli (including damaged cells) in an effort to initiate the healing process. You are likely familiar with some of the symptoms of acute inflammation, such as those caused by insect bites. The area begins to turn red and quickly becomes inflamed. This type of inflammation typically involves the rapid discharge of white blood cells to the affected area. This type of bodily response is not at all negative and can sometimes save your life when you are infected by harmful external agents.

The type of inflammation I'm referring to, which is responsible for a variety of chronic maladies, is the type that occurs in your body silently over time. This type of inflammation sneaks up on you like a thief in the night and can only be detected by an increase in the inflammatory signals produced by your immune system when you have a severe infection or are recuperating from an injury. It also manifests its ugliness when it begins to cause a variety of problems in the body. Many individuals and physicians easy make the mistake of treating the symptoms of these diseases rather than chronic inflammation, which is the root cause of the issue.

"But what causes this chronic inflammation?" You may inquire. Indeed, this is our livelihood. The foods we consume and the way we live all contribute to the obesity, metabolic syndrome, and other diseases that plague our society, and it all comes down to inflammation.

Let us examine the effects of the chemicals in many of the foods we consume today on our bodies and immune systems after they have seduced our taste buds and entered our intestines.

You are formidable. Close your eyes and visualize light permeating the environment. This is a secure location. Here is your secure haven. You are currently residing in a lovely bubble. It is plush, cushiony, and utterly relaxing. Consider the sounds of your respiration and my voice as you drift off to sleep. Imagine these sounds as a river moving upstream slowly and methodically. In this sphere, you're as light as a leaf. There is no constraint. You feel merely light and airy. And even as you experience weightlessness, you continue to sense the force field of the surrounding luminous energy. Permit the ship to transmit you up the river. Listen to the sounds of nature that you are surrounded by in this sacred location. Open your inner vision.

Observe the grandeur around you. You are in a secure location. You embody the sun. You are one of nature's most potent entities, and you are currently performing the functions of the sun. You radiate brightness. You radiate brilliance and beauty. Your emanated light is therapeutic, restorative, and potent. You feel the energy accumulating within you, and you sense the power of the light consuming those negative thoughts. You are unique, and this light was created to flourish. Imagine an orb of light ascending a river. You are this luminance. This luminance is you.

Maintain your respiration. Take a single breath at a time. Inhale thoroughly. Exhale gently. Maintain this cadence.

There is no reason to hurry. You are not rushing. You have time on your side. This is a transformative occasion. Take a full breath in. Feel your thorax expanding as you inhale. Allow the oxygen to settle in your stomach. Now let go of the breath. Relax. You're doing very well. As thoughts begin to form in your consciousness, resist them not. But don't engage them either. Stay in your luminous cocoon. Now proceed upstream along the river. Imagine the bubble you're in as you ascend. As you ascend above the water, you are no longer borne by the river's current. You move in the same direction as the watercourse without being affected by it. As you distance yourself from the river, you distance yourself from the material world. Your capsule is positioned directly above the river. It shifts an imperceptible parallel line to the river.

As you approach the first river bend, I want you to repeat after me: "I release myself from the physical, mental, and emotional burdens that bind me to my fears and pain." I tear down every memorial I've erected in recognition of a negative past experience. I renounce any vows I have taken out of anger, shame, or grief that have prevented me from forming positive relationships with others. I am releasing any mental fists of unforgiveness that exist in my heart. I wish to be liberated from my anxieties, self-doubts, and inability to advocate for myself. I am consciously and subconsciously deciding from this point forward to prioritize my opinion and perception of myself over those of others. I reclaim my freedom of choice, and I choose to be better, stronger, and more assured today. Today, I awaken my inner colossus. I choose to empower myself today. Today, I am easily making a commitment to myself: to accept myself for who I am, to embrace every facet of myself, and to refuse to treat myself with disdain by judging my abilities by the standards of others. From now on, my standard is myself.

Take a deep breath now. Hold it for several seconds, then let go. Feel the energy percolate up in your stomach as you speak these words. You have now established the framework for this guided exercise and are prepared to move on to the next phase. Maintain even and regular respiration. You are undergoing a transformational voyage. There is nothing but good on the other side. So let go of anxiety and concern. These feelings are not permitted in this area. Your bubble has approached the river's turning point. You are surrounded by clouds, and you have no notion what lies beneath them. But rather than worrying that you will collapse, you should focus on the fact that the cloud is there to catch you. Keep this idea in mind as you commence your descent. You are not physically decreasing in size. You have just entered the following realm. Accept the procedure. Maintain your respiration.

You are alright, and you will feel even better in a few moments.

Therefore, it is possible that these words you are gazing at have nothing to do with you. It is possible that the individual who used this word was projecting their own insecurity onto you. This may not immediately easy make you feel better, but it will help you understand the origin of this word. It has nothing to do with what you could have or should have done. Because it is about the other person, you should not be coping with this issue in the first place. Therefore, as you prepare to send this message, embrace the truth that you have just discovered. The word does not refer to you. You do not resemble this word at all.

Now, if the word you are confronted with is something from your subconscious, in the sense that you have chosen to use it to characterize yourself, then the issue is perspective. You must cease viewing yourself through the lenses you currently employ. Low self-esteem is fueled by self-doubt, and both contribute to a decline in confidence. The truth is that this term you have used to describe yourself is not accurate because you are comparing yourself to a nonexistent model. You are a robust, courageous, and mighty individual. The more you begin to identify with these sentiments, the more you will recognize their truth. As a result, for this final exercise on this plane, you will eliminate every negative conception you have developed about who you are. No matter how small it may be, you must let it go.

To begin this procedure, you must identify every negative word that describes your persona or character. Imagine them as desiccated leaves falling to the ground. Take a deep inhalation after holding these leaves in suspension. Use this breath to purge out any lingering negative emotions caused by these words. Give a forceful exhale. As you exhale, visualize the foliage floating away. This text should not be confined to the crystal space. You must

47

eliminate them. Release them. They are falsehoods, and as with all lies, they have no substance when compared to the truth.

Chapter 5: Effective Ketogenic Diet Menu Plan Strategies

As I explained in the previous chapter, there is a high likelihood that your keto diet will fail if you don't have the correct perspective when you begin.

If you are not mentally prepared for your weight loss journey, you will likely fail at the majority of other regimens. Do not presume that this only applies to ketogenic diets.

Due to your lack of mental preparation, you may experience emotional lulls that could prompt you to abandon the keto diet sooner rather than later.

Fortunately, if you have the right mindset, you can employ several strategies.

The correct "attitude" is essential for weight loss. It is not negotiable. There is no way to evade it. Before proceeding, I recommend that you attentively read Chapter 10 .

The following are three essential strategies for beginning and maintaining a ketogenic diet.

Brief Note

Changing to a ketogenic diet is uncomplicated. Seriously.

You would be enthusiastic when beginning any regimen. You would be anxious to get started because you are aware of the many benefits. After seeing the results other people achieved, you are anxious to give it a try.

The problem is not starting up. It is wonderful to be energized, enthusiastic, and prepared. Compliance is the issue.

For this reason, you need the proper mindset and food preparation techniques. Take special note of the following.

Concentrate on fat-rich foods you enjoy.

Avocado is one of the high-fat foods commonly recommended to individuals who are just commencing a ketogenic diet.

Evidently, avocado is the "typical suspect" in this instance. It is high in lipid and fiber content. Why not cherish it?

If you don't like avocados, it may taste like consuming a piece of wax. It requires some alterations.

The majority of individuals combine avocado with another sustenance. Either they use it to easy make guacamole and serve it with Mexican cuisine, or they use it to easy make ice cream.

You are now aware that ice cream is not permitted on a ketogenic diet. This refreshment is loaded with lactose-containing milk and sugar. Consequently, all you have is a simple avocado.

There is a means of avoiding this. Focus on oily foods that already possess the flavor profile you enjoy. In other words, stay with what you already know.

Load up on specific foods, such as pork rinds and other salty, fatty treats, if you already consume them. Now is not the time to acquire new preferences.

As I explained in Chapter 10 , the key to effectively adjusting to keto and maintaining it for an extended period of time is displacement, not replacement.

When you search out new tastes or attempt to retrain your taste buds to accept them, you are replacing.

Never convince yourself that you are replacing your previous diet. No. You are replacing. A flawed strategy.

Eventually, something will unravel, and you will return to your previous dietary habits. Focusing on oily foods that you already enjoy is a superior strategy.

The good news is that they already exist. Many individuals who do not follow a ketogenic diet consider these items to be sinful indulgences. They believe these foods should be ingested infrequently.

Your wish will be granted if you adopt a ketogenic diet because you can consume these foods daily. Isn't that wonderful news?

Focus on hearty foods with flavor profiles that you enjoy.

Try to feel content for an extended period of time.

Consider your sustenance selections throughout the day. Ask yourself, "Will consuming more of this type of food easy make me feel fuller for longer?"

If you don't understand where I'm coming from, recall the times you used to snack on pears. Apples are a nutritious and light snack, but you will inevitably feel famished again after consuming them. This occurs due to the sugar content of pears.

If you substitute chocolate bars, confectionery bars, or cookies for apples, the same principle applies, but on a much larger scale. Your fluctuating blood sugar levels encourage you to consume munchies throughout the day.

After adopting a ketogenic diet, be mindful of your food selections. Because your body processes the oil in your system differently when you replace the apple with, for instance, a teaspoon of cream cheese, you will feel full for a longer time. When you consume fatty foods, your body and brain send a variety of appetite signals.

Therefore, it is imperative that you choose your refreshments carefully. As a snack, consume macadamia almonds rather than anything else. This item is saturated with oil, and your body is aware of it. You experience prolonged abundance.

Chapter 6: Bulletproof Diet Overview

Bulletproof nutrition is a diet that enhances the mental and physical performance of humans. The bulletproof diet seeks to provide you with a healthy body and a clear mind in order to attain the highest level of health. This regimen encourages daily consumption of adequate calories. It also suggests that 60% of the diet should consist of healthful fats and 20% of protein. The remaining twenty percent should be vegetables.

According to research, many prevalent diets are detrimental to human health. The focus of these investigations was biochemistry and human performance. The results revealed that men's modern eating habits sapped their vitality and made them irritable. Additional investigations revealed that many dietitians suffer from low immunity.

The bulletproof diet's primary caloric sources are:

Fats -- Experts regard unsaturated fats to be the "healthy" type of fat; therefore, it is best to consume foods rich in unsaturated fats. Additionally, saturated lipids can be beneficial. High density lipoprotein cholesterol (or HDL), the beneficial cholesterol that prevents heart disease and other cardiovascular diseases by increasing HDL cholesterol levels, has been shown to be increased by saturated fats.

Cow, goat, and lamb provide saturated lipids such as butter, lard, and ghee. Additionally, cocoa butter, coconut oil, and avocado oil are excellent sources of healthy lipids.

Protein is essential for the development of robust bones and muscles. Consider consuming grass-fed red meats, such as beef, lamb, and other red meats. White meat and eggs from free-range poultry are excellent protein sources. It is also worthwhile to contemplate shellfish such as shrimp and clams.

Vegetables - Since the majority of vegetables are low in calories, you can consume as many as you desire. Because they are abundant in vitamins, minerals, and essential nutrients, green verdant vegetables are highly recommended.

Broccoli, spinach, kale, and asparagus are among the healthy vegetables. Carrots, sweet potatoes, and succulents are all permitted. However, they should not be ingested excessively due to their high carbohydrate content. Other -- Fruits should be consumed in modest amounts; daily consumption of 1 to 2 cup of chopped fruit is sufficient. It is possible to consume a reasonable quantity of coffee, tea, and cocoa to keep your mind sharp and stimulated, despite not being prohibited from doing so.

The failsafe diet discourages consumption of carbohydrates. The diet plan must exclude grains like wheat, rice, and porridge. There are no legumes, dairy products, or seeds on the food list.

Uncooked food is more nutritious than cooked food. The bulletproof diet prioritizes raw ingredients. If food preparation necessitates cooking, the finest options are baking or steaming. These methods will preserve the majority of a food's nutrients without modifying its flavor. Poaching and boiling are acceptable culinary techniques.

Chapter 7: Boost The Effectiveness Of Your Ketogenic Lifestyle With The Following Modifications.

I'm not going to tell you an untruth. Changing one's diet can be extremely difficult. It will require a considerable amount of exertion. It requires considerable concentration and fortitude.

And if you want to adhere to a diet and keep the weight off permanently, you will need to prioritize consistency.

There are, thankfully, modifications that will allow you to convert your keto diet into a keto lifestyle. This is actually the key to any weight loss program.

If you view diet as merely a means to reduce a few pounds here and there, you will likely regain the weight. The only variable is time.

Conversely, if you view your weight loss system as a gateway or transition point to a different lifestyle, the weight will likely remain off. This is how it operates.

Consider the following modifications. I do not expect you to master all of these on your first attempt. Usually, it takes some time to become accustomed to them, but if you give them sufficient attention and significance, they will ultimately become second nature.

Chapter 8: The Bulletproof Diet

In order to be successful on this diet, you must first determine how you will consume and what you can eat. Therefore, I will outline the guidelines, as well as the foods you should consume on a daily basis and those you may want to consume less of. Then, I shall inform you of the foods you must avoid. After that, we'll delve right into some delicious, diet-friendly bulletproof recipes!

Before we discuss what you will consume, you need to understand the unique proportion guidelines for this diet. The Bulletproof Diet, unlike many other diets, does not require you to cease eating when you are still hungry.

In fact, you are encouraged to consume as much food as you desire at each meal and to stop eating when you are no longer famished. The disadvantage is that you will have to avoid snacking, but if you can consume as much as you want in one sitting, you probably won't be hungry between meals.

If you feel like eating less than the required amount during a meal, do not compel yourself to consume more. Your body will let you know when it requires sustenance and when it feels sluggish.

Yes, you will consume a great deal of fats on this diet, but don't worry! They are healthful fats that will fuel your body and keep you alert and focused throughout the day. For a moment, let go of all your negative beliefs about fat and imagine a world in which you never had to worry about that pesky word again. This is the Bulletproof universe.

70% of your daily caloric intake should originate from fats.

This is the second most crucial component of the Bulletproof Diet. Similar to the majority of other dietary plans, protein is an essential component. However, the Bulletproof Diet recommends that you consume 20% of your daily calories as protein.

Non-Carbohydrate Vegetables

Twenty percent of one's daily caloric consumption should come from non-starchy vegetables. This may seem like a low number, but in actuality, your plate will consist primarily of vegetables due to their low calorie content. Remember that you'll be coating them in sea salt and grass-fed butter, so they'll be delicious!

Fruits and Carbohydrate-Rich Veggies

These will only account for 10 % of your daily calorie intake. If you want to lose weight on this diet, you may want to avoid fruits and carbohydrate vegetables six days per week and allow yourself one day to consume one serving of each.

For the first two weeks of the Bulletproof Diet, your breakfast will consist of this Bulletproof Coffee blend. If you are a woman, an athlete, or someone who will lose over fifty pounds of weight, you should consume a small amount of protein with your coffee. If you are expectant or trying to conceive, you may wish to prepare this recipe for No-Coffee Vanilla Latte.

After completing the initial fourteen-day phase, you will enter the maintenance phase, during which you can consume a protein- and fat-rich breakfast every morning with your coffee. Here you will discover some of those recipes. Consuming at least some protein will help you avoid cravings.

Now, after breakfast, you will abstain from food until luncheon. That means no more snacks or caffeine. Intermittent fasting is beneficial for your health because it allows your body to eliminate old cells in the intestines and stomach lining, as well as reduce fat.

Evening Meal

The evening meal should consist of approximately thirty grams of Bulletproof-friendly carbohydrates and vegetables. Once per week, consume between one hundred and one hundred fifty grams, preferably on Bulletproof Fasting days. If you're trying to lose weight, you may want to reduce your carbohydrate intake each night, as this will accelerate your weight loss.

On carbohydrate re-feed days, women typically require approximately 6 00 grams more carbohydrates than males. As long as they adhere to the rest of the diet's principles, pregnant women should limit their carbohydrate consumption each night.

If you eat a large dinner, you will sleep easier at night. If you have difficulty sleeping, consume some protein, such as whey protein concentrate, before bed. You can add the concentrate or fresh honey to the No-Coffee Vanilla Latte before going to bed.

Rapid Protein Digestion

Once per week, you will restrict your daily protein intake to no more than twenty-five grams. If you notice that you are losing muscle mass or experiencing other undesirable side effects, increase your protein intake until you find a healthy balance.

Soup With Ginger And Sweet Potatoes

6 C. Water

1 tsp. Salt

4 Tbsp. Butter

4 Tbsp. Coconut Oil

6 C. Cubed, Peeled Sweet Potatoes

3 C. Carrots, Sliced

2 Tbsp. Grated Ginger

1. Heat the oil in a pan and add the sweet potatoes through the ginger. Sauté for 1-5 minutes.

75

2. Add the water and simmer for thirty minutes covered.
3. Add the salt.
4. Place into a food processor and blend until smooth.
5. Add the butter and blend once more.

Bulletproof Pleasant Cupcakes

easy make Ingredient List:

- Dash of Salt, Himalayan Variety

- 12 Eggs, Large in Size and Separated

- 4 teaspoons of Vanilla, Powdered Variety and Mold Free

- 2 teaspoon of Cocoa Powder

- 2 tablespoon of Flour, Sweet Rice Variety

- 12 Tablespoons of Erythritol

- 12 Tablespoons of Xylitol

- 24 Ounces of Chocolate, Dark Variety

- 2 1 Sticks of Butter, Unsalted Variety and Grass Fed Variety

Instructions:

1. The first thing that you will want to do is preheat your oven to 350 degrees.
2. While your oven is heating up line two muffin pans with muffin liners.
3. Add your Erythritol and xylitol into a blender and pulse until finely ground. Set this mixture aside for later use.
4. Then use a small sized saucepan and add 4 cups of water into it.
5. Simmer over low to medium heat.
6. Next add in your chocolate and butter into a large sized bowl.

7. Place this bowl directly over your water and allow to heat up until completely heated through.
8. This should take at least 20 minutes.
9. Remove from heat and allow to cool slightly before serving.
10. Use a stand mixer and add in your Erythritol mixture, dash of salt and egg yolk.
11. Blend on the medium to high setting until your mixture is thick in consistency.
12. This should take at least 5-10 minutes.
13. Fold your egg mixture into your melted chocolate mixture.
14. Add in your vanilla, cocoa powder and flour.
15. Fold again to incorporate.

16.   Use a separate bowl and add in your egg whites.
17.   Beat with an electric mixer until soft peaks begin to form.
18.   Add into your Erythritol mixture and continue to beat until peaks begin to form.
19.   Add in your chocolate mixture and fold again until combined.
20.   Spoon at least ½ cup of your batter into your muffin cups.
21.   Place into your oven to bake for the next 45 to 50 minutes.
22.   Remove and allow to cool for the next 10 minutes before transferring to a cooling rack.
23.   Enjoy whenever you are ready.

Smoked Salmon And Eggs

easy make Ingredient List:

• 8 Tablespoons of Ghee, Grass Fed Variety and Fully Melted

• 2 teaspoon of Dill, Fresh

• 8 Eggs, Pastured Variety and Poached

• 1 Cup of Salmon, Smoked Variety and Wild Caught Variety

• Dash of Salt, For Taste

Instructions:

1. First heat up your ghee in a large sized skillet placed over medium heat.

2. Once your ghee is fully melted add in your dill and cook for at least 60 seconds.
3. Remove from heat.
4. Place your smoked salmon among two serving plates.
5. Top off with your poached eggs and cooked dill.
6. Season with a dash of salt and serve right away. Enjoy.

Delicious Protein Smoothie With Bulletproof Coffee

Ingredients

2 scoop of chocolate protein powder, or of choice

2   cup of brewed Bulletproof Coffee, chilled

2 cup of ice

2 cup of almond milk, or of choice

2 chopped organic banana, frozen

2 tablespoon of raw honey

2 tablespoon of cocoa powder, unsweetened

Directions

1. Gather all of the listed ingredients, add them into a blender and blend until the mixture is smooth.

How To Prepare Simple Chicken Curry

Easy make List of Ingredients

40 Grams of curry spice

100 Grams of tomatoes

2 00 Grams of fat free yogurt

250 Grams of mushrooms

100 Grams of onion

140 Grams of cucumber

500 Grams of chicken

4 Cloves of garlic

First, you must easy cut all of your ingredients into segments of comparable size. After chopping the ingredients, you should position a saucepan over low heat. Spray the pan lightly with a low-calorie culinary spray or olive oil.

After the pan has attained a boil, the onion should be added and gently stirred for one minute. Then, incorporate the cucumber and the poultry. Be sure to thoroughly combine the ingredients before adding the garlic.

Now is the moment to add tomatoes and curry seasoning. All the ingredients should be stir-fried for three minutes. If you observe that the vegetables are beginning to stick to the pan, add a splash of water. Add the mushrooms near the end of the cooking process and continue to stir the ingredients until the mushrooms are nicely browned.

If the meat begins to turn a golden-brown hue, you should remove the pan from the heat and add diced tomatoes and stock. Be sure to simmer for thirty-six minutes before removing the pan. In conclusion, consume two teaspoons of fat-free yogurt.

Easy make Easy make Easy make

Bulletproof Matcha Cappuccino

Ingredients:

- 2 tbsp unsalted butter
- 2 tbsp sugar-free maple syrup

- 2 cup hot water
- 2 tsp matcha green tea powder

Instructions:

1.
   Add all the ingredients to a blender and   mix   until   smooth.

2. Pour into a glass and enjoy!

Bulletproof Chai Latte

Ingredients:

- 2 cup fresh strongly brewed black tea
- 2 tbsp MCT oil
- 2 tbsp unsalted butter
- ½ tsp cinnamon powder
- ½ tsp ginger powder
- 2 tsp sugar-free maple syrup

Instructions:

1.

   Mix all the ingredients in a blender until smooth and serv in a glass.

Italian-Style Gratin

4 basil leaves

2 tsp heavy cream

2 tsp grated pecorino

2 Mozzarella balls

1   pinch Fleur de sel

2 Small eggplants

2 00 g Sausage meat

20 tbsp. to s. olive oil

6 tbsp tomato puree

1 tsp sweet pepper

2 garlic cloves

Preparation of italian-style gratin:

Wash the eggplant and easy cut it into narrow slices. Drain the salt in a colander. In a pan with oil, brown the sausage flesh and set aside. Brown the eggplants and sauté them in olive oil in the same skillet.

Peel and mince the garlic cloves. Chop the basil leaves. Combine tomato puree, chile, garlic, basil, and a small amount of water. Slice the provolone.

Preheat the oven to 220 degrees Celsius (th. 7-8). In a baking dish, arrange eggplant in a single layer.

Cover with tomato sauce, crème fraîche, sausage, and mozzarella. Commence layering these ingredients. Finish with pecorino cheese. Bake in the oven for twenty minutes.

easy cut

Brazilian Truffle-Style Coconut Balls

5 tsp. Butter

1 tbsp. Coconut oil

5 tbsp. powdered sweetener

15 cl Unsweetened condensed milk

130 g Grated coconut

25 hazelnuts

Preparation of Brazilian truffle-style coconut balls:

1. Faites fondre la veille sur feu doux l'huile et le beurre.
2. Mélangez avec le lait concentré, 100 g de noix de coco râpée et l'édulcorant.

3. Remuez le temps que se forme une pâte homogène.

4. Réservez cette pâte une nuit au réfrigérateur.

5. Le lendemain, enrobez chaque noisette d'2 cuil. à s. de la pâte à la noix de coco, formez des boules.

6. Passez la noix de coco restante rapidement à la poêle et roulez chaque boule dedans.

Eggs Scrambled With Spinach

Ingredients:

4 cloves garlic, minced
4 red onions, diced
1 teaspoon dried oregano Pinch of salt,
pinch of pepper

12 eggs
1000 grams ground beef
4 cups spinach
4 tablespoons coconut oil

1. Trim spinach, chop coarsely and then set aside.

2. In a large skillet, heat coconut oil and saute onion and garlic until golden.

3. Add oregano to the skillet and mix ingredients well.
4. Season the mixture with salt and pepper.
5. Add the ground beef to the skillet and continue to cook for about 5 to 10 minutes.

6. Add spinach to the skillet and cook for another 1-5 minutes or until wilted.

7. Add beaten eggs to the mixture, stir, and continue to cook for about 4 minutes or until set.
8. Transfer scrambled eggs on a plate and then serve immediately.

Tuna Salad

Ingredients:

2 red bell pepper, diced
4 teaspoons fresh rosemary, chopped 1
cup parsley, chopped
Pinch of salt
Pinch of pepper

400 grams tuna fillet
8 cups mixed salad greens

2 tablespoons capers, rinse
1 cup freshly squeezed lemon juice
2 red onion, chopped finely

Place tuna in a saucepan, cover it with water, and add a teaspoon of salt.

Bring the water to a boil, then simmer the tuna for approximately 5 to 10 minutes.

Put the tuna on a plate and allow it to settle down. Then, crumble it.

In a basin, combine tuna, capers, and onion.

Whisk together lemon juice, olive oil, and a sprinkle of salt and pepper in a salad bowl.

Toss the salad greens with the oil and lemon juice mixture before serving.

Before serving, add the tuna mixture to the basin and gently toss to combine.

Peanuts Added To Iced Bulletproof Coffee

Ingredients:

2 cup newly fermented coffee

- 4 tbsp sans sugar maple syrup
- Whipped cream for topping
- 4 tbsp squashed toasted peanuts

- 2 tbsp MCT oil
- 2 tbsp butter
- 4 tbsp unsweetened cocoa powder

Instructions:

1.

Except the whipped cream and peanuts, add every one of the fixings to a blender and interaction until smooth.

Pour the beverage into a glass, whirl a few whipped cream on top and embellishment with the peanuts.

Soup With Cashews, Ginger, And Butternut Squash

Ingredients:

2 -inch piece fresh ginger, grated

4 tsp. ground cumin

4 tsp. ground cinnamon

2 large butternut squash

2 can (2 8 oz.) coconut milk

2 c bone broth or veggie stock

12 carrots, chopped

2 c raw cashews, chopped

Directions:

1. Combine all ingredients and easy cook for 1-5 hours on low in a slow cooker or on the
2. stovetop on low heat, stirring regularly, for 1-5 hours.
3. Blend to a smooth
4. consistency before serving.

This Vegetable Curry With Rice

Ingredients:

6 T coconut oil

8 leeks, sliced

4 cans (2 8 oz. each) coconut milk

4 zucchini, diced

6 limes

2 sweet potato, peeled and diced

2 small butternut squash, peeled, seeded and diced

4 T Thai green curry paste

Directions:

1. Heat oven to 350 degrees F. Melt 4 T of the coconut oil and mix with 4 T of the
2. Thai green curry paste.
3. Toss the sweet potato and squash in this mixture, and
4. then put it all in a roasting pan.
5. Season with salt and roast for about 60 minutes.
6. To begin the sauce, melt the remaining 2 T of coconut oil in a fry pan. Cook the
7. leeks until softened and golden.
8. Stir in the remaining 8 T of the curry paste and
9. easy cook for a few minutes. Add the coconut milk and a splash of water and simmer.

10. Add the roasted vegetables along with the zucchini. Simmer for 25 to 30 minutes.
11. Stir in the juice from the limes and serve over rice.
12. Thoroughly rinse white rice before cooking to be bulletproof.
13. Rinse and rinse
14. until the water's clear.
15. Then cook as usual.

Keto Chosolate Avosado Mousse

Ingredients

- 5 tbsp Cacao powder, raw

- 1/2 cup Coconut milk (full-fat)

- 2 packette Stevia sweetener, powder

- 2 avocado(s) Avocado • 2 scoop Protein Powder, Bulletproof Collagen

Instructions

1. Chill ripe avocado for 1-2 hours prior.

2. Add avocado to your blender, along with chocolate and protein powders, followed by the coconut milk.
3. Add sweetener of choice (optional).
4. 8 . Put the lid on and blend for 20 seconds then rest for 20 seconds in intervals until mousse reaches silky consistency.
5. Transfer to bowls and add your favorite toppings! See "Notes" below.

Citrus Conut Energy Bites

Fresh lemon

Ingredients

• 1 tbsp Bulletproof Brain Octane Oil

1/2   cup Coconut, shredded, unsweetened (organic)

• 2   tbsp Fresh lemon peel (zest) (optional)

• 4 bar Collagen Protein Bars, Fresh lemon cookie

• 1   tbsp Honey, raw (room temperature)

Fresh lemon

Instructions

1. Using a food processor or a fork, finely crush the bars.
2. Add in the honey and Brain Octane, blend into a mixture.
3. Fold in the shredded coconut and distribute evenly with a spoon or spatula.
4. Using a spoon to scoop, mold each bite into the shape and size of a ping-pong ball.
5. Sprinkle a little coconut and fresh lemon zest (if desired) on the top to finish.
6. Refrigerate for one hour before serving.
7. Makes 5-10 fresh lemon coconut energy bites, lasts up to 6 days if continuously refrigerated in a sealed container.

Wraps Of Spicy Bacon

Ingredients:

½ teaspoon chili powder
1/2 teaspoon ground black pepper 24
slices bacon
4 avocados, peeled and pitted.

½ teaspoon garlic powder Hot sauce

Method:

1. Wrap each avocado slivers with bacon and place them in a lightly oiled baking sheet.

2. Season the wraps with garlic powder and black pepper.

3. Bake the baking sheet at 450 °F for 35 to 40 minutes.

4. Transfer the wraps on a platter and then sprinkle with hot sauce and chili powder before serving.

Sautéed Atlantic Salmon

1 teaspoon cumin seeds

1 teaspoon fennel seeds

1 teaspoon black mustard seeds

1 teaspoon fenugreek seeds

1 teaspoon nigella seeds

2 teaspoon sea salt

1 cup coconut oil

2 leek, well washed and thinly sliced (optional)

4 celery stalks, thinly sliced

4 carrots, finely chopped

10 spears baby asparagus, trimmed and finely chopped 2 can coconut milk, well shaken

2 head bok choy, cored and chopped

8 wild sockeye salmon fillets 2 tablespoon Bulletproof Brain Octane oil

1. In a medium pot, combine the leek, celery, sarrot, and araragu and cook, stirring frequently, for approximately 48 minutes, or until softened.
2. Add coconut milk, bok choy, salmon, cumin, fennel, mustard seeds, fenugreek seeds, nigella seeds, and sea salt.
3. Cover and simmer for 1-5 minutes, or until the vegetables are tender and the fish is cooked through.

4. Drizzle the coconut oil and Brain Octane oil over the dish.

Eggs Poached With Sautéed Greens

Ingredients:

-4 Eggs, Poached

-4 Tbsp. of Almonds, Sliced Finely

-1-5 Cups of Kale and Collards, Freshly and Washed

-4 Tbsp. of Butter, Unsalted and Grass Fed

-Dash of Sea Salt For Taste

Directions:

Fill a vessel of medium size with about an inch of water. Prepare your mixed greens over a medium heat. Cook your vegetables until they are tender. Empty out your water.

Next, add the butter and stir the greens until they are completely coated. Remove heat from your vegetables.

Sprinkle your greens with salt and nuts, then swirl to combine. Add poached eggs to the dish and serve immediately.

Delicious Grapefruit With A Hint Of Cinnamon

Ingredients:

-Sprinkle of Nuts, Organic and Your Personal Choice

-2 Grapefruit, Medium In Size and Organic

-Dash of Cinnamon, Organic

Directions:

1. Slice your grapefruit in half using a serrated knife.
2. Then slowly loosen the sections of the grapefruit as carefully as possible.
3. Next place your grapefruit pieces onto a baking sheet.

4. Easy make sure that you sprinkle each slice with a generous amount of cinnamon and finely chopped nuts.
5. Set your oven to broil and place your grapefruit slices into the oven.
6. Broil for the next 5 to 10 minutes or until the tops of the grapefruit slightly brown.
7. Remove from oven and serve immediately.

Salad Of Artichokes And Bacon Lard

Ingredients

½ cup chives, chopped

½ cup warm bacon fat

6 tablespoon apple cider vinegar

2 tablespoon honey

4 cups artichoke in oil

2 head of cos lettuce, finely sliced

10 radish, sliced

Salt and pepper to taste

Method

1. Warm the bacon fat in a small sauce pan and add the honey, vinegar and chives.
2. Combine the artichoke, radish and lettuce in a bowl.
3. Pour over the dressing and mix well.
4. Serve immediately.

Kale Pesto

Ingredients

2 cup virgin olive oil

1 cup basil leaves

Salt and pepper to taste

2 pound of kale

½ cup raw almonds

Juice of half a lemon

Method

1. Lightly cook the kale in boiling water and transfer to food processor.
2. Add the rest of the ingredients and blend, keeping the mixture fairly course.

Sardine Salad

Ingredients:

8 cups mixed salad greens

4 teaspoons capers, rinsed

1 cup black olives, chopped

450 grams sardines in tomato sauce

2 tablespoons apple cider vinegar

4 tablespoons olive oil

Method:

Whisk olive oil, tomato sauce, and apple cider vinegar together in a basin, then set aside.

In a large basin, combine salad greens, black olives, and capers.

Add the sardines and dressing to the basin, and then toss them together gently.

Serve without delay.

Rack Of Roasted Lamb With Celery, Cauliflower, And Fennel

Ingredients

4 cups sliced cauliflower

2   American rack of grass-fed lamb -
about 8 chops

Sea salt

4 cups sliced celery

2 tablespoon ghee

2   tablespoon freshly chopped thyme,
sage, oregano, rosemary and turmeric

4 cups sliced fennel

Directions

1. Preheat your oven to 350⁰F. Evenly
   rub the ghee over the lamb chops and
   diagonally score top fat.
2. Sprinkle salt and chopped herbs over
   the dog.

3. Place your veggies in a pan and place the lamb, the fat-side facing up, on top.
4. Bake until the lamb gets to 150 ^{0} in the thickest sections, roughly 10 to 15 minutes.
5. Get the oven to low broil and leave to cook for three more minutes for the skin to crisp.
6. Leave some for tomorrow's lunch.

Strawberry Crunch Beverage With Fewer Carbs

Ingredients

2 tablespoon of chia seeds (optional)

1 cup of frozen organic strawberries

Roughly 4 tablespoons of almonds

2 cup unsweetened vanilla almond milk

1 teaspoons cinnamon

Directions

Put all the ingredients in a blender or magic bullet (if you are a smoothie connoisseur, the magic bullet is a blender you should consider).

Blend to your desired consistency.

Sweet Potato Smoothie

Ingredients:

8 ice cubes

2 pinch cinnamon

2 large sweet potato, peeled and cubed

2 carrot, sliced

1/2   cup raw almonds

1-2   cups coconut water

Directions:

1. Combine all the ingredients in a powerful blender or food processor.
2. Pulse for 1-5 minutes until smooth and well mixed.
3. Pour the smoothie in glasses and serve it right away.

Smoothie With Avocado And Chocolate

Ingredients:

2 1 cups coconut milk

2 tablespoon erythritol

2 ripe avocado, peeled and pitted

4 tablespoons natural cocoa powder

Directions:

1. Mix all the ingredients in a blender and pulse until smooth and creamy.

2. Pour the drink in glasses and serve it as fresh as possible.

Brussel Sprout Squash

Ingredients:

20 brussel sprouts

2 squash, peeled, deseeded and chopped into chunks

Method:

1. Lightly steam brussell sprouts.
2. Push ingredients into juicer.
3. Easy make sure to alternate ingredients as they being pushed into the juicer so the mixture is an even consistency.

Smooth Avocado

Ingredients:

- 1/2   of an Avocado

- 4 tablespoons of avocado oil

- Handful of Ice

- 2 cup all natural Almond milk

- 1/2   cup Almonds

Method:

1. Put all the ingredients into a blender.

2. Start on a low speed and increase to a high speed.

3. Stop blending when all ingredients are fully blended.

Easy Cut Easy Cut Pomegranate-And-Hazelnut Slaw With Cabbage

A generous dash of fresh chopped coriander

2 organic pomegranate

2 teaspoon sea salt

2 tablespoon organic fennel seeds

Organically grown purple cabbage

2 organic carrot

8 cups of organic fresh and tender spinach

10-15 radishes 1 cup of chopped organic hazelnuts

How to go about it:

1. Using a sharp knife, easy cut spinach very finely.

   2. Thereafter cook cabbage and spinach separately for 10 to 15 minutes respectively.
3. Then let both cool and place them in a large bowl.

4. Add a teaspoon of salt, toss spinach and cabbage.

5. Use your fingers for the purpose and squeeze them lightly for about 2

143

minute easily making them even more tender and soft.

6. In order to easy cut carrots into thin strips use a potato peeler.

7. Scrape the radish and easy cut it into long and thin slivers.

8. Add radish and carrots to the cabbage and spinach mix and give it a toss.

9. Now take the rubies from the pomegranate, hazelnuts, and chopped

coriander and fennel seeds and add them to the bowl.

10. Add salt to taste and prepare the dressing for the salad.

11. Take 2 tablespoon apple cider vinegar, 6 tablespoons extra virgin olive oil, 1 teaspoon organically prepared mustard, juice of organic pomegranate and whisk it all in a bowl.

12. Add salt to taste.

13.   Place the salad on each plate and add to it a generous drizzle of the dressing.

14.   Enjoy and get ready to gather all the compliments coming your way.

15.   With all the cutting and chopping involved, the entire procedure would take around 80 to 90   minutes and serves 8 to 6 people.

Smoothie Made From Raspberries And Cabbage.

Ingredients:

- 2 cup frozen raspberries
- 2 tablespoon lemon juice
- 2 cup shredded red cabbage
- 2 cup almond milk
- 2 tablespoon MTC oil
- 2 tablespoon upgraded collagen

Directions:

1. Place all ingredients into a food blender.
2. Process until smooth and blended thoroughly.
3. Serve immediately.

Bulletproof Elixir

Ingredients:

- 1 tablespoon cacao powder
- 1 teaspoon vanilla powder
- 2 0 stevia drops
- 4 tablespoons upgraded vanilla protein powder
- 2 cup warm green tea
- 2 tablespoon coconut oil
- 2 tablespoon grass-fed butter or ghee
- 2 heaped tablespoon chia seeds

Directions:

1. Place all ingredients into a food blender.
2. Process until smooth and creamy.

3. Serve immediately in a chilled glass.

Bulletproof Rice

Ingredients:

1 lemon, sliced

8 tablespoons ghee, divided

Sea salt to taste, if desired

4 cups white rice, cooked

4 lemons, freshly squeezed

1-5 tablespoons MCT oil

Preparation:

In a large saucepan, melt 1-5 tablespoons of ghee over low heat. Add cooked rice and thoroughly combine. Add a pinch of salt and about three-quarters of the freshly strained lemon juice, if desired. Stir frequently and heat the ingredients for up to five minutes, or until they are heated. Stir in the remaining butter for an additional minute. Remove from heat and finish with the remaining lemon juice and a slice of lemon.

Avocado Caprese

½ of a cup of balsamic vinaigrette

2 of an avocado that has been easy cut out in chunks

1 ball of mozzarella cheese

2 0 grape tomatoes

1. Easy make small chunks out of your mozzarella cheese so that they are the same size as the chunks of your avocado.
2. Easy cut slits into the grape tomatoes so that the juice comes out slightly.
3. Mix all of this together in a large bowl.

4. Coat with balsamic vinaigrette.
5. You can eat this as soon as you easy make it but it will be more flavorful if you let the mixture marinate overnight.